THE GIFT WITHOUT BORDERS:

My Healing Journey

SHERRY HARDT

Dedicated to:

God (Higher Power)

and

Kristy Parker

who was fearless, supportive and stood
by my side during my healing journey

Contents

PROLOGUE

When I was in my teens and early twenties, I wondered what I would be doing in the year 2000, as did many of my peers. This was a time to look forward to and wonder what advancements we would be experiencing.

Would I be in a highly successful career? Would I be happily married and have children? What would the world be like?

On April 14, 2000 at 3:15 p.m., I got a phone call at work from my Doctor which would change everything for me. I was in my office when the call came in.

An urgent voice said, please wait for the Doctor. The Doctor came on the line and announced in a serious tone, "we found an aneurysm in the brain and it is centered in the middle of your brain."

Suddenly my brain was on overload and unbelief. Time slowed to a crawl. All my senses went into over-drive. It was almost as though I was frozen in time.

Within moments of getting THE NEWS, I remembered that Norman Cousins had healed himself of an incurable disease with laughter. I had been studying the book, The Power of Your Subconscious Mind by Dr. Joseph Murphy, for several years. I thought this was as good a time as any to put it into practice.

I also rested on my connection with God (Higher Power), and the knowing that prayer is very powerful and that with belief, faith and expectation, miracles can happen!

This is my story.

Chapter One -
THE NEWS

"Every adversity, every failure, every heartache carries with it the seed of an equal or greater benefit."
                                    -Napoleon Hill

It was late afternoon on April 10, 2000 and I was working at Heritage Hardwoods in Southern Indiana where I was the Human Resources Manager. I was in charge of hiring the staff, handling employee relations' issues, developing and facilitating training, and oversight for payroll and benefits for two hardwood veneer plants which sat side by side.

I had an office with one door into the main office, which was filled with sunlight most days, and one door into the warehouse where the product was generated by the staff.

Many times I would glance out the window into the warehouse to see a forklift zooming by very close to my window. The President had thought about this and had a shatterproof window put into the office. My office was decorated with wood paneling, wood floors and a wooden desk, as were all the other offices, since we were in the hardwood veneer business.

This particular day I was scheduled to present training on the employee handbook to all the employees. As I prepared for the meeting, I looked down on the page of materials and the words became blurry – the letters didn't mean anything. It was like looking at a jumbled foreign language.

Suddenly, there was a hole in the middle of the words and the other letters around the hole were fuzzy. None of this made any sense! I became dizzy and struggled to plop down in a chair before the floor came up to meet my face.

As I took a breath to stabilize myself, numbness seeped up my right arm and spread around my mouth. Someone came into the training room and asked about upcoming classes.

I struggled to respond, my brain told me what to say, yet different words came from my mouth – very much to my surprise! I was able to give the person a training calendar and pretend all was normal. After all I was at work as the Human Resources Manager, so I couldn't let anyone know my head was reeling and my brain was not functioning correctly.

I was glad that no one could actually see the malfunctioning that was going on inside my brain. However, I knew I couldn't teach the class and had to go home before my health got worse or more symptoms starting showing up.

I called my boss and told him that I had a migraine headache and could not teach the training class. He was sympathetic and told me to put a note on the door canceling the class and not to worry about it.

I logged onto the computer and typed up a note that the class was canceled. I posted the cancellation notice on the door of the training room while my head and stomach were reeling.

I shuffled out to my car, struggled and squinted to see the road and managed to drive myself home, but knew I would need to seek medical attention once this episode passed. I felt too bad to consider going to the hospital or doctor and dealing with their questions and bright lights. I had migraines in the past and knew that if I could just get home in a dark room and pass out, the headache would go away.

My real concern was with the new symptoms of numbness in my arm and around my mouth and my brain not functioning right. The first available appointment with my Internist was several days later. I told the Doctor about the episode of blurred vision, migraine headache, along with the numbness in my arm and around my mouth and the difficulty speaking my thoughts. I also told him about the previous migraine headaches I had experienced for several years on a sporadic basis which made me ill to the point that I had to go home, throw up and be in total darkness.

The Doctor immediately ordered an MRI for the next day. I took my friend Beth with me as the Doctor seemed very concerned.

The MRI was quite an experience; it was like being enclosed in a tight dark tunnel with loud clanging noises. I started to hyperventilate but then used self-hypnosis with peaceful scenes to slow my breathing down and make it through the procedure. I made a plan to not ever go through this again. It was almost as bad as having a migraine.

Two days later, which was Friday, April 14, 2000, I got a call at work from my Doctor's office around 3:15 p.m. The Nurse said in an urgent voice, please wait for the Doctor. My Doctor came on the phone and immediately said he wanted me to see a Neurologist on Monday. He wanted to know when I could go.

I felt confused, alarmed and asked why I needed to see a Neurologist. The

Doctor announced in a serious tone; "Oh, well we found an aneurysm in the brain and it is centered in the middle of your brain."

Suddenly my brain was on overload and unbelief. Time slowed to a crawl and all my senses went into overdrive. It was almost as though I was frozen in time.

I said, "Whoa Back Up. What exactly is an aneurysm?"

This was a stall tactic while my body shifted into hypervigilance and my mind was searching memory banks for the word aneurysm and the meaning.

The Doctor explained that an aneurysm is like the tube inside a bike tire that has a bubble in it and that I needed to go see a Neurologist immediately – preferably Monday. I guess he meant it could swell up, leak or explode and this was an urgent situation.

I went into shock, felt over-whelmed by this information but agreed to the appointment with the Neurologist on Monday.

I was at work in Southern Indiana and the Doctor was in his office in Kentucky. However I could feel his urgency and concern across the phone line. He just wanted me to stop talking and agree to the appointment. After I agreed to the appointment, I sat in this unreal moment of THE NEWS. Everything remained in slow motion.

I wanted to go home and talk to family and friends and get some support. Fortunately the warehouse workers left at 3:00 p.m. on Fridays so only the Secretary was there. However, my next thought was of the company Family Fun Day I was in charge of the next day.

We were hiding 600 Easter eggs for the employees and their families, plus having a cookout and games for the children to play, which included beanbag toss, guess how many jelly beans in the jar, go fish, pet the real bunny and meet the Easter Bunny. There was no time for this challenge in my life! What the heck was going on? Why was this happening now?

Chapter Two -

MY
DECISIONS

"The capacity for hope is the most significant fact of life. It provides human beings with a sense of destination and the energy to get started."

-Norman Cousins

Faith is being sure of what we hope for and certain of what we do not see.

-Hebrews 11:1

As I sat in my office and let THE NEWS wash over me. I had been diagnosed with an aneurysm in the middle of my brain. A memory came to me very strongly that Norman Cousins had healed himself with laughter from an incurable disease and I could do the same.

Norman Cousins was a longtime editor of the Saturday Review, a global peacemaker, receiver of hundreds of awards including the UN Peace Medal and nearly 50 honorary doctorate degrees.

In 1964 following a very stressful trip to Russia, he was diagnosed with ankylosing spondylitis (a degenerative disease causing the breakdown of collagen), which left him in almost constant pain and his doctor told him he would die within a few months. He disagreed and reasoned that if stress had somehow contributed to his illness (he was not sick before the trip to Russia), then positive emotions should help him feel better.

With his doctors' consent, he checked himself out of the hospital and into a hotel across the street and began taking extremely high doses of vitamin C while exposing himself to a continuous stream of humorous films and similar "laughing matter". He later claimed that 10 minutes of belly rippling laughter would give him two hours of pain-free sleep, when nothing else, not even morphine could help him.

His condition steadily improved and he slowly regained the use of his limbs. Within six months he was back on his feet, and within two years he was able to return to his full-time job at the Saturday Review.

During the time of his illness, Norman Cousins maintained his sense of humor, despite the dire prognosis that his illness was rapidly disintegrating the connective tissue of his spine and he was told he could die in a few months.

Norman Cousins sensed that his

mind and his spirit each had a role to play in making his body well again. He had respect for the medical community but also respect for the human body's ability to heal and regenerate itself. He felt that emotions were a powerful contributor to health. (Anatomy of an Illness by Norman Cousins).

I had been studying the book, The Power of Your Subconscious Mind, by Dr. Joseph Murphy for several years. In this book, Dr. Murphy states, "your subconscious mind is the builder of your body and is on the job twenty-four hours a day. You interfere with its life-giving pattern by negative think-ing."

In the ten minutes I sat in my office trying to make sense of the an-eurysm diagnosis, I quickly made the decision to put into practice the ideas of Norman Cousins' healing himself with laughter. I also decided that I would tap into my spiritual foundation and beliefs and maintain a positive outlook, find joy in my life, live in each precious moment, appreciate everything around me, continue living my daily life doing normal activities and surround myself with people who would be supportive.

Once I made the decision of how I would handle my diagnosis, I told the Plant Manager and the President about the aneurysm and told them to keep it quiet and that we could continue with the Easter Egg Hunt and Family Fun Day event. They willingly agreed to keep my diagnosis private, which filled me with relief.

I called my daughter Holly and my good friend Kristy and told both of them about my diagnosis and asked if they would help me get through the Family Fun Day event. I knew they would be there for me and not freak out about the diagnosis.

They were both up for the challenge and stepped right in to help with the event. I blocked out the diagnosis as if it didn't exist. I stayed in the moment enjoying the children laughing as they found the Easter eggs, threw bean bags, grabbed a hot dog, played with the live bunny and visited with the Easter Bunny (the Plant Manager). The event was very successful and I was relieved when it was over.

After the Family Fun Day was over, Kristy and I decided to go to Thunder over Louisville, which is the kick-off celebration two weeks before the Kentucky Derby. We parked about 10 blocks away since 650,000 to 700,000 people typically attend this event. We went into a local liquor store and decided to purchase four bottles of Tequiza (our favorite drink) to celebrate the fireworks and the kick off to the Derby.

We walked a few blocks, sat down and watched the crowd. We laughed at all the coolers on wheels going down the street while a large shadow engulfed us as a Stealth fighter plane flew overhead. Slowly we walked a few blocks at a time, finding something funny to laugh about in the crowd, until we finally made it to the event.

When we got to the riverfront, we experienced all the smells of a carnival; smoky sausages, onions and peppers frying, tantalizing pizza smells, frothy beer and sugary elephant ears. I stayed in the moment and enjoyed the excitement of the crowd waiting for the fireworks to begin. This isn't just your ordinary fireworks event! During the day there are airshows to get the crowd ready for the fireworks display, which begins around 9 p.m. It is one of the largest annual fireworks displays in North America. The fireworks are synchronized to a soundtrack piped through a tower of speakers. Also the Second Street Bridge is closed the day before the event so that fireworks can be set up on the bridge.

During the event people line the banks of the Ohio River in Louisville,

Kentucky and also across the river in Jeffersonville and Clarksville, Indiana to see the airshows and the fireworks. Others watch from boats on the river or at docks along the riverfront. The boaters pay money to charities for the position they get in the river.

Eight 400-foot barges located on both sides of the Second Street Bridge launch the fireworks, while more fireworks are launched from the bridge. It is a spectacular free party and attendance is approximately five times that of the Kentucky Derby horse race at Churchill Downs.

The weather was gorgeous and we had a truly wonderful time as I stayed in the moment and just enjoyed being alive and experiencing the crowd, music, and laughter with my friend Kristy and the beautiful fireworks over the water.

Chapter 3 -
MY JOURNEY- WHAT IS MY REALITY?

"Be empty of worrying.
Think of who created thought!
Why do you stay in prison?
When the door is so wide open."

— Rumi, The Essential Rumi

"Our beliefs control our bodies, our minds, and thus our lives..."

— Bruce H. Lipton, The Biology of Belief: Unleashing the Power of Consciousness, Matter and Miracles

But on Monday, reality started to show up. This was a scary time for me but yet I didn't really believe I had this aneurysm in my head. How are you okay one day and have something bulging in your head the next day? My daughter Holly went with me to see the Neurologist. As tears streamed down my face, the Neurologist confirmed that the MRI showed an aneurysm in the middle of my brain.

My children were 20 and 17 at the time and we were very close as I was a single parent from the time they were 5 and 7. I couldn't imagine not getting to see them be successful in life, see them get married, and have families of their own.

The Neurologist, Dr. Hodes, told me, "I will know you more than your closest friends as we go through this process."

He took my health history and when he got to addictions, I said none and my daughter laughed. She said, "oh yes she is addicted to coffee."

The doctor confirmed that he didn't count that as an addiction. My daughter's comment made me laugh because she definitely thought I was addicted to coffee since I always reached for a cup the moment I got up in the morning.

Dr. Hodes gave me two options; one was surgery which included cutting into my skull to examine the aneurysm. The Doctor would then make a decision in the moment of what to do with the aneurysm.

The other option was a new procedure where they would go up through the groin into the brain with a small camera. Dye would be injected into the brain. This would allow for mapping of the brain to see where the aneurysm was located. After this procedure we would then decide what could be done about the aneurysm.

Since the second option didn't involve an incision on the head, I decided I would take this option. I definitely wanted to avoid cutting on the head or the brain and losing my hair.

I told Dr. Hodes I wanted to put off the procedure for a month because I had a vacation planned to go to Florida. My good friend Kristy and I had already planned a trip to visit my brother and sister-in-law, Keith and June in Florida on the following week.

Dr. Hodes agreed to delay the procedure for a month and told me that I could do anything I wanted to do except skydiving or parasailing. I felt relieved that I had time to get away from the diagnosis for a while and be in my favorite place, the sunny beaches of South Florida.

I called my Mom and Dad to give them THE NEWS and my Mom's immediate response was, "I don't think the aneurysm is there". I held onto this statement tightly as my mantra, through the next month. I felt deeply in my soul that this must be true as my Mom is a Nurse, so she should know. This statement was definitely a gift that kept me thinking positively about my situation. She was confirming my thoughts and belief that the aneurysm did not exist.

I had been attending a series of workshops at my church as a volunteer mentor in the Care Ministry. This ministry is where lay people receive 50 hours of counseling training to walk side by side with people who are going through a crisis in their life and support the person with prayer and counseling until the crisis passes.

All of the sudden, I was the one who needed someone by my side to walk through this crisis with me. I turned to this group for comfort and prayer. They were very supportive and immediately began to pray for a healing. Again I did not believe in the aneurysm. I believed in maintaining a positive attitude, so I worked each day to present a positive attitude to those around me and had faith that I would be healed.

I continued to think about how Norman Cousins healed himself of an untreatable disease with laughter, and that the patient must become involved in the healing process. I looked for something to laugh about each day. I would end my day by watching an episode of the Friends show because no matter how many times I watched the show, it always made me laugh.

Most of the time I was able to show a positive attitude to the world but occasionally I felt my world shaking and sadness would start to drift in. I would immediately shift my focus to let go of negative thoughts by going into meditation, finding something to laugh about, going into self-hypnosis, going for a walk in a peaceful place in nature, talking to a trusted friend, or praying to keep my positive outlook that everything would be okay.

When I was reminded of the aneurysm, I would start playing a mental movie in my mind where I viewed myself happy and healthy walking on the beach on a beautiful sunny day and put my focus on that instead of the aneurysm. I would get into all the feelings and emotions of being at the beach with no worries or concerns.

I knew basketball players and golfers visualize the end result (getting the ball in) to improve their game. So I believed in visualizing myself well to bring about that outcome.

In a research study, psychologists at the University of Chicago took three groups of basketball players. Group One practiced foul shots each day for thirty days. Group Two was instructed to "imagine" shooting foul shots each day for thirty days. Group Three was instructed to do nothing.

When tested, Group One (practicing shots) improved 24 percent. Group Three (doing nothing) had no improvement. Group two, the group that only imagined shooting foul shots, improved 23 percent yet did not physically touch a basketball.

Therefore, I visualized myself happy and healthy each day, as I knew it was a very powerful practice to see and feel healthy and vibrant.   I knew that the subconscious mind could not tell the difference between real and imagined.

Chapter Four -

THE GIFT WITHOUT BORDERS

"The greatest healing therapy is friendship and love."
-Hubert Humphrey

"Healing is simply attempting to do
more of those things that bring joy and
fewer of those things that bring pain."

-O. Carl Simonton

My good friend, Kristy, was a bright light in my life during this life challenge. She agreed to continue our planned vacation even though there was a chance of my "brain exploding". These were my words of humor to ease talking about the situation.

When I mentioned this, she took it in stride and said she would write down anything that happened out of the ordinary with regard to my brain. Believe me she took this job seriously!

I met Kristy at the Louisville Gas and Electric Company, the local utility company, where we both worked in the 1990s. I was chosen to fill in for her on a work project while she was on vacation. I had a feeling right away that we would be close friends.

We both knew there was something more to life than working hard all our lives and we were searching for this answer. We continued our friendship after I left the utility company in 1996.

Through all our ups and downs in life we have maintained an acceptance of each other without any judgment, which makes our relationship very special and unique.

Kristy didn't treat me any different after the aneurysm diagnosis. She gave me the gift of love and support and a vacation without borders. It was up to me to pick anything I wanted to do and she would help make it happen.

With heightened emotions, great joy and expectation, I began to make a list of fun activities for us to do with no worries about the future.

We left for our trip on an early Saturday morning in April, when crocuses were just beginning to sprout their heads in Kentucky. We decided to fly from Louisville to Orlando, Florida and then drive to Palm Beach Gardens, Florida, which is close to West Palm Beach, where my brother Keith lives with his wife June.

We decided to visit my brother and sister-in-law because they would help fulfill my dreams before the surgery. We arrived in Orlando and discovered we had to ride a shuttle over to get our rental car. We had booked the car online and knew we had gotten the best deal possible at the Dollar rental agency.

To our surprise the car was a little compact without automatic windows or automatic doors in a concrete metal color. It didn't look like it had much get up and go. We immediately named it the Roach Coach and it stuck for the rest of the trip. We loaded up our big suitcases and set out for Palm Beach Gardens – not quite sure of our directions but knew we needed to head South.

After about two hours on the road we decided that we probably should call my brother Keith to get directions to his home. To my surprise, I didn't have his phone number or address information with me but I managed to remember his phone number.

I used Kristy's new cell phone to call my brother's phone number and I got his answering machine. I started to leave a message and asked Kristy what her phone number was – she looked at me with embarrassment as she said, "Uh, I'm not sure, and I just got this phone."

I asked her if she had written the number down and she said no. We both busted out laughing; here we were on the vacation without borders to visit my brother and yet we did not have his address and couldn't leave a message since we didn't know Kristy's cell phone number. This was so funny to us that we had to immediately pull the Roach Coach over.

Once we were under control, I came up with a brilliant idea. I had written down Kristy's new cell phone number in my business calendar, which was at home on my kitchen table. I called my son Chris and asked him to look up Kristy's cell phone number in my calendar. When Chris listened to my request, he exclaimed, "Aren't you with her?" I had to explain that yes I was with her but she did not have a clue as to what her cell phone number was.

Chris called my brother Keith and let him know we were on our way but needed directions. We continued on our way and another hour passed and we had not heard from Keith. I tried his number again from the cell phone and a voice came on and said the number was out of service.

I couldn't believe it so I asked Kristy to stop at the next rest stop. I went inside and used the pay phone and after dialing the number a lady came on and said the number was out of service. What were we going to do since we didn't have directions?

I called my son again and checked the phone number with him and he said it was the correct number. He had left a message an hour before for Keith to call us on Kristy's cell phone. We decided to keep heading south. I thought surely he will call us as he was expecting us and knew what time we were scheduled to arrive.

Finally my brother called about 30 minutes later and gave us directions. I wondered if we had already passed the exit he was talking about but we continued on looking for the exit. After another 20 minutes we decided to get off of the road and ask for directions.

We discovered we were in Lake Worth, Florida, which is about 20 miles south of Palm Beach Gardens, Florida. While we were trying to figure out if we were close to our destination, a man who looked homeless came towards our window.

We became apprehensive. He seemed incredibly tall and was disheveled looking. I said, maybe we should give him money and he will give us directions and go away. He took the money and the directions he gave us included going west. We asked which way that meant and he told us to go left away from the ocean.

We finally arrived at the hotel about a half hour later and went into the room to unload our suitcases and the drinks we had brought with us. Kristy went to move the car while I worked on getting the room set up. My focus was on getting the Tequiza chilled as quickly as possible. I made several trips to the ice machine to get stocked up. I put the bottles in the sink and piled ice on top and around the bottles – we had it down to a science and knew the drinks would be iced down within 12 minutes.

I didn't realize that the hallway door locked when Kristy went down to move the car. I was playing music and could not hear her banging on the hallway door. She started throwing rocks at the window trying to get my attention.

Suddenly my brother and sister-in-law walked up to Kristy's embarrassment. She had never met them before so she choked back a laugh. She asked them if they were coming to see me and told them she was my traveling companion and trying to get back into the hotel. When they all threw rocks at the window I looked out and saw them yelling to open the hall door.

My brother Keith and sister-in-law June were ready to help with the fun things to do list. They followed my lead and didn't make a big deal of the diagnosis. I had created the list of fun things to do with great exuberance and joy, and after showing it to Kristy we decided to add piercings and tattoos to the list just to see my brother's expression.

He looked at the list and said in a serious tone, we can do everything on the list except I don't know where to go for piercings or tattoos. We busted out laughing so he knew we were just having fun with him.

Keith and June suggested we go to a Hammerheads baseball game, which wasn't on the list but sounded like fun. After all, we had escaped the cold weather in Kentucky and were now enjoying being outdoors in the warm sunshine. We enjoyed the game and saw an advertisement on the fence for a bar named Uncle Micks and thought we might check it out later.

The next day started out with a gorgeous beautiful sunny morning. I decided to get up early and go down by the pool and let Kristy sleep in. When Kristy came down to the pool, she asked me if I had cleaned up the bathroom before coming to the pool.

I laughed and said, "No way I'm on vacation." She realized the room attendant must have come in and cleaned the room while she was asleep. I busted out laughing. Kristy was in shock that she slept through someone cleaning the room.

We decided to take a walk on the beach. The ocean was aquamarine and you could see all the way through it to the sandy floor. We walked a couple of miles until we came to the Jupiter Beach Resort Club. We decided to blend in with the hotel guests at the Resort and enjoy the pool. A gentleman sunning himself nearby offered to bring us towels.

After a while we decided it was time to eat but the service was very slow and we had to complain to the manager to finally get some food. We hadn't eaten anything all day and had some Dirty Monkey drinks when we first arrived at the resort.

A monstrous headache over-whelmed me and we had to walk all the way back to our hotel which was at the other end of the beach.

Kristy became very concerned about my headache considering the aneurysm diagnosis. She said we needed to get back to the room and write everything down.

I said, hey Kristy, maybe the headache is from only eating a muffin, being out in the hot sun all afternoon, drinking the Dirty Monkey and not eating lunch until 3:00 p.m."

When we finally got back to the room, after walking on the beach 4.5 miles, I took some aspirin and lay down with ice on my head. Within 30 minutes I was ready for more adventures since the headache was gone and my brain was still intact.

That night we wanted to go out and have some fun so we asked June about bars in the area. She told us whatever you do don't go to Uncle Micks. We drove around for a while and couldn't find any place to go so we looked at each other and said why not try Uncle Micks.

We walked into this dark dungeon of a bar with a dance floor on one side and pool tables on the other. We decided right away that we wanted to play pool, so we set up a table.

Two guys came up and watched us play and then asked if they could play with us. They introduced themselves as Mike and Tom. They told us they had just gotten off work at the local Home Depot. We decided to pair up with the guys and play 8 ball.

We were wearing our short white shorts and having a great time playing pool, laughing and joking. I don't know how in the world it happened but each time I was trying to miss the 8 ball – I managed to get the 8 ball and the cue ball in the pocket to end the game, actually 3 games in a row! This night was so much fun and full of so much laughter that the aneurysm and the headache were totally forgotten.

Keith and June decided to take us on an adventure to South Beach for two days of sun and fun. They were very generous in offering to show us a good time and told us they had reserved a suite for us on the beach.

When we arrived in Miami they took us to a very special Cuban restaurant called Versailles where the food was delectable and the service was impeccable. Next we went to our hotel in South Beach. The first thing we noticed was that everyone was on their cell phones no matter where they were; on the beach, in their cars and even in the pool.

We went to Lincoln Street and had dinner outside at Next, and saw a famous musician sharing dinner with his dog sitting up at the table. All this while a homeless lady sat across from the restaurant watching us eat. At the end of our meal she approached us for our leftovers which we promptly gave to her.

We walked up and down the streets looking in the windows and experienced an eccentric brand of art.

Next we went to Mangos where the girls danced on top of the bars. The Latin dance floor was packed with amazing dancers who dipped and swirled intensely with the music.

We ordered drinks several times and no matter what it cost, no matter what bill was given, we never saw any change. Apparently this was part of the culture in Mangos. We enjoyed being a part of the immense energetic crowd that consumed this nightclub.

We walked around downtown going in jazz clubs and looking in the store windows in our dresses and heels and were amazed at all the people that were wandering the streets until 2:00 a.m.

After South Beach we drove over to Naples, Florida to visit my parents and grandparents. While in the pool, my mother introduced me to her friends and they asked if this was the daughter with the "aneurysm".

While I was ignoring the aneurysm, apparently my Mom was telling all her friends. They expressed sympathy and best wishes and I quickly changed the subject and presented my positive outlook and talked about how much fun I was having in Florida.

After leaving Naples behind, we headed back to Orlando. We stayed at the Renaissance Inn. We had two telephones in our room, which included one in the bathroom. We went to Pleasure Island at Disney World and started dancing and talking to people in the street. We met Mike and Mike from

Chicago who were dancing on the spinning dance floor.

We hung out and danced under the stars in a pretend New Years' Eve celebration at Pleasure Island. We had so much fun just being in the moment and everyone was so friendly.

Kristy has always been directionally challenged so when she got in the car to drive us back to the hotel, I wasn't sure what would happen. We were leaving Pleasure Island at Disney World and had to get back to the hotel. It was totally amazing because for the first time ever she drove straight to the hotel without asking directions and without having to turn around!

The vacation was far beyond my dreams. We did something fun and exhilarating every day. We enjoyed the simplest things and laughed about everything.

The feeling I had was, why not try anything and everything because what did I have to lose. This was a very freeing way to look at life with joy in every moment.

I knew the surgery would be waiting for me when I returned but I didn't have to think about it or put any focus on the diagnosis. So I consistently kept my focus on fun and away from the aneurysm. I actually got to the point that I did not believe in the diagnosis although my Doctor and Neurologist were convinced it was there based on the MRI. I was beginning to create my own reality where the aneurysm did not exist!

Our joy in the moment brought all these fun experiences and fun people into our life. However, as the trip was ending, I had to consider what was next with regard to my brain. I concentrated on pushing away any thoughts of the aneurysm and maintaining positive thoughts. I continued to play the mental movie of being happy and healthy at the beach and put my focus on that instead of the aneurysm.

I spent time in nature with appreciation for all of the good things in my life. I found something to laugh about every day to continue getting my laughter fix.

Chapter Five -
THE
PROCEDURE

"There are only two ways to live your life.
One is as though nothing is a miracle.
The other is as though everything is a miracle."
-Albert Einstein

"True imagination is not fanciful day-dreaming; it is fire from heaven."
-Ernest Holmes

The week before the procedure I had to go for tests and blood samples were taken to prepare for the procedure. At times I could feel the seriousness coming back into my mind about the aneurysm as I moved through all the steps the medical profession required to prepare for the procedure.

But once again I would move my thoughts to a memory of how much fun we had at the beach or I would do self-hypnosis or go into prayer to get relaxed about the procedure.

I went to the hospital for the procedure early in the morning on May 18, 2000. Kristy was there along with my parents and my daughter Holly and my son Chris, who had come home from college. I had signed my living will and prepared myself for the procedure.

The Doctor and four assisting staff members escorted me into the operating room. I felt the hush of the room and seriousness started to weigh down on me in this sterile room, as this was a new experimental procedure. I prayed that all would be well when the procedure was complete. I readied myself to let go and just be in the moment without fear.

I was awake during the procedure because I had to help the Doctor during the surgery by holding my breath when the dye was infused into the brain. I could see several computer screens of my brain on my left side during the procedure. However without my glasses on, I really could not make out much on the screens.

Once the procedure was complete and while I was still lying on the bed in the operating room, the Doctor came over and whispered in my ear that the aneurysm was not there but that he wanted to see me in his office the next day.

Yes it was GONE! The exhilaration inside me popped like a cork in a bottle, allowing joy for the beauty of life to expand. Wow! Here was my miracle and the Gift Without Borders which was given from tapping into the healing love of God (Higher Power), the healing love of friends, family, prayer community; my belief in the power of the subconscious mind to heal, and using the healing tools of meditation, prayer, self-hypnosis, visualizing positive healthy images, being in joy and laughter each day and my faith and belief that I only saw myself as healthy and happy.

However I went home feeling like someone had punched me really hard in the stomach and with a monstrous headache, the worst ever. I took some aspirin and used self-hypnosis to go into sleep.

Not knowing exactly what the Doctor would say the next day, my parents went with me to the appointment. As we met with the Doctor he let me know that all the pathways in my brain were clear and open and that I was totally released from his care to go live my life.

I did not ask questions about his medical opinion of what had happened with the aneurysm in my brain. It was clearly there at the time of diagnosis but not there a month later. Just as I did not research my diagnosis and find out what could have happened, I did not look for medical answers to why or how it could have disappeared. I knew and felt in my soul that through prayer, loving support, and joy, I was given the miracle of health and I was not looking back. I just wanted to go forward and live life more consciously and in celebration for what life offers.

On Sunday, two days after the procedure, I was able to attend the Care Ministry retreat to complete my training as a mentor. All the mentors were happy for me. It was wonderful to connect with God (Higher Power) in gratitude during this spiritual retreat surrounded by nature in the beautiful woods of Southern Indiana.

After I was diagnosed with the aneurysm, I would look at pictures first thing in the morning and the last thing at night, of times when I was happy and healthy so that it would be easy to feel just like the picture. This helped me focus on feeling healthy and normal and helped me disregard my diagnosis.

So you might wonder what created the aneurysm. As I looked back on the year right before the aneurysm, it was clear that my thoughts were of worry and depression as I had experienced many life changes. My grandparents and parents had moved away. My children were ready to be launched out into the world. I had broken off a nine-year significant relationship and I had a new job as a Human Resource Manager with a lot of responsibility.

Yes our thoughts and feelings aren't just thoughts and feelings, they seep down into the subconscious mind and anything held in the subconscious mind is considered true and will be created in our world.

If we have continual worry, sad or depressed thoughts, we create that environment in us and around us. The same is true for happy, positive, joyful thoughts as experienced during my journey to health.

I was fortunate that I had learned about how to tap into the power of the subconscious mind two years before I had the aneurysm, from reading Dr. Joseph Murphy's book, The Power of the Subconscious Mind. So I had the knowledge to produce miracles and now was the time to put this knowledge to use!   I made a pact with myself to live life in the moment with much laughter, joy and adventure, while knowing all is well.

According to Marilyn Mandala Schlitz, PHD, when you go from frustration to joy, 1400 chemical changes happen in the body.

Per Dr. Oz and Dr. Roizen, a research paper published online in September 2013 in a journal of the American Heart Association, shows that even for people dealing with heart disease (the number one killer of adults in the US), a positive outlook means living longer and stronger, or as they say, living younger.

Ralph Waldo Emerson said, "Man/Woman is what he/she thinks all day long."

Chapter Six-
The
Creation
Formula

"You can't get to the finish line unless
you start."

Sherry Hardt

"Never finish a negative statement, re-
verse it immediately and wonders will
happen in your life."

"Just keep your conscious mind busy
with expectation of the best."

Dr. Joseph Murphy

So you might want to know the formula I used to heal myself of an aneurysm, sell my house in two days and have it be a cash deal, move across the country to my dream location in Florida while keeping my current job, manifest retirement money from a job I worked in for six years in the 90's, sell my car in two hours and have $5,000 cash in my hand, and be in the highest possible joy.

I tapped into the creativity that creates worlds when I aligned with positive energy and God or Higher Power, which is present everywhere and in everything. Once you tap into this energy and believe that what you desire can come for you, YOU have the capacity to change your world and do things you never thought were possible.

It's always our decision about how we see a challenge, how we feel about it and whether we think we can do anything about it. But if we decide to do it alone it is much harder to get there. We most likely will not experience the surprising ease that comes about when we access the energy that creates worlds. As we are asking for the change we desire, it's important to release all doubt and feel the joy that our desire is coming to us.

You may have heard of the Law of Attraction and know that it basically means that like attracts like. Just like magnets attract, your thought will attract to you what you are thinking about whether it is a positive thought or a negative thought. These ideas have been known for a long time and even expressed in the Bible. Here are some references to the power of the law of attraction.

Therefore I tell you, that whatever you ask for in prayer believe that you have received it, and it will be yours.
                                                    Mark 11:24

"Whatever you hold in your mind on a consistent basis is exactly what you will experience in your life."

-Anthony Robbins

"What you radiate outward in your thoughts, feelings, mental pictures, and words, you attract into your life."

-Catherine Ponder

The first step is to know that your thought is creative. What you think about will be created in your experience whether it is what you want or not. Everything in your world now you created by your thought. Keep your attention on what you want and let thoughts of what you do not want go. By being aware of your thoughts and keeping them focused on what you want, letting go of the rest, you will get there!

Knowing that you are the creator of it all will change your life. You can relax and decide what you would like to experience and then focus your thought accordingly. You can make a change at any time by letting go of the old thought while creating new thoughts and getting clear about what you desire.

Beliefs are crucial to bringing your desire into your world. So believe that you can have it, know that it is coming, expect it to come; then relax and allow it to come to you. A very clear knowing that you can have what you desire is the power that brings the desire into your world.

Many times we take our health for granted until we aren't healthy and then we experience a great desire to again be healthy. It's important not to focus on the illness but instead focus on the health that you desire.

Get into the feelings of happiness and joy that your desire is on its way. Don't worry or have doubts, as this will slow down or stop the process. When you are light about it or in joy and laughter it will come to you quicker as you will be aligning with all of creation.

As you are focusing on your desire, you may receive inspiration to take an action. This action will not be like trying to make something happen which is push energy. Instead be playful in thinking about your desire and don't worry about how it will come about.

It might be that you get the idea to call someone, go get a massage, take a wellness class, or someone may show up and give you information that you feel you should act on.

When I had my house on the market and pictured living in Florida, I suddenly got the inspiration to schedule the moving truck, even though my house hadn't sold yet. This was energy movement and belief towards my goal of living in Florida, so I scheduled the moving truck for Memorial Day weekend, which would give me the long weekend to move. However, within a couple of weeks I called the moving company to change the date to an earlier date as my house had sold in two days.

So you start with a desire of what you want and you think about this desire in a positive way, you talk about your desire, you imagine it, you pretend that you have it, and you play with the idea of having it. You play a mental movie of it happening while you feel the feelings of having it, and these feelings and thoughts become familiar or a habit to you and then you relax and allow the desired result into your world.

While in this process you might suddenly change your thoughts to a new desire, so let go of your previous desire and begin the creation process with this new desire.

Allowing it to come to fruition is holding yourself in a state of relaxation knowing that what you desire is coming. Let go of will power or trying to make it happen, just stay in a knowing that what you want is already on its way to you.

The Creation Formula-

Here is my example of using the Creation Formula for the desire to have a healthy body and release the aneurysm.

Thought/Desire: I want to be healthy, happy and live a joyful life.

Belief: Yes it can happen! I believe it can happen. I can be healthy. The aneurysm does not really exist.

God/Higher Power/Divine Source: Daily stating affirmative prayer to align with God energy while knowing that I have a perfectly, healthy body just as I had always experienced up to this point.

Example: It is my divine right to be healthy and I know that my connection to God energy or Higher Power heals all weakness.

All the cells of my body, work together for the good of my body.

I am healthy and happy now, right in this moment. I am so thankful and grateful now that I am well.

Master Mind: I told people about my diagnosis who I knew would support me through this health challenge by being positive, helpful, loving, praying for me, and treating me with respect and understanding.

Inspired Acton: Maintaining positive and joyful thoughts. Finding things to laugh about. Watching Friends episodes each day. Staying in the moment and experiencing joy and appreciation in the moment. Going for walks in nature. Asking my Doctor if I could go on my planned vacation to Florida. Creating a list of fun things to do.

Looking at pictures first thing in the morning and the last thing at night of times when I was happy and healthy so that it would be easy to feel just like the pictures. This helped me focus on feeling healthy and normal and helped me let go of my diagnosis.

Vision: Playing a mental movie of doing fun things, laughing, and being healthy and happy at the beach. I got into the feelings of happiness that my desire could come true.

Expectation: By aligning with God, Source or all that is and maintaining my vision of health, it will happen! Excitement, it can happen soon!

Reality: Approximately one month after the diagnosis of the aneurysm in my brain, it was totally gone. I was told

I had a healthy brain and released to go live my life.

Aligning with God or Higher Power, thought, belief, gratitude, joyful feeling, healthy vision, knowing and expectation formed into Reality!

Chapter Seven -

THE POWER OF OUR THOUGHTS AND BELIEFS

"A person's health isn't generally a reflection of genes, but how their environment is influencing them. Genes are the direct cause of less than 1percent of diseases: 99 percent is how we respond to the world.

-Bruce Lipton

"Understand that the right to choose your own path is a sacred privilege. Use it. Dwell in possibility."

-Oprah Winfrey

Sherry Hardt

We have the power to heal with our thoughts and beliefs

In 2002, researchers at the Houston VA Medical Center and at Baylor College of Medicine found that a common type of knee surgery known as debridement, surgical excision of dead, devitalized, or contaminated tissue and removal of foreign matter from a wound, to be no more beneficial than a placebo surgery. A placebo is a substance, drug, or procedure that has no therapeutic effect, used as a control in testing new drugs or in this case used to measure the effectiveness of the knee debridement.

The patients were divided into four different groups and no one knew who would get the surgery or who would not get the surgery, not even the doctors. Two groups got the surgery and two groups did not get the surgery.

The Doctors would go into surgery and open an envelope and then find out if they were doing the surgery or not.

The patients who did not get the knee debridement surgery were given a fake surgery that included three incisions made in the same location as in the real knee surgery. The staff then played a video as though they were doing the surgery and passed the instruments and talked as though the surgery was taking place. They stayed in the operating room the same amount of time as though the surgery was taking place.

"I was initially very surprised," Dr. Bruce Moseley, an orthopedics professor at Baylor, told United Press International. Dr. Mosley performed both the real and placebo surgeries in the study and stated, "I could not imagine anybody suggesting that anything we do in surgery would be beneficial from a placebo effect. I associate placebo effect with pills."

Throughout a two-year follow-up, the 180 patients in the study were unaware whether they had received the "real" or placebo surgery. Patients who received actual surgical treatments did not report less pain or exhibit better functioning of their knees compared to the placebo group. In fact, periodically during the follow-up, the placebo group reported a better outcome compared to the patients who underwent the debridement surgery.

One participant who benefited from Dr. Moseley's placebo knee surgery said, "The surgery was two years ago and the knee has never bothered me since. It's just like my other knee now."

Dr. Mosley's study, was a randomized, double-blinded, placebo controlled clinical trial, and the results were published in the New England Journal of Medicine, which showed that the placebo group experienced resolution of their knee pain solely because they believed they got surgery.

Negative thoughts can create symptoms of illness

The nocebo effect is when a negative expectation of a phenomenon causes it to have a more negative effect than it otherwise would. Both placebo and nocebo effects are presumably psychogenic but also produce measurable physiological changes as well as changes in the brain, the body and behavior. (Wikipedia)

In Lissa Rankin, M.D.'s book, Mind Over Medicine, she states that one study showed that 79 percent of medical students report developing symptoms suggestive of the illnesses they are studying. Lissa experienced this herself during her first year of medical school as she was studying the many ways the body can be impacted by illnesses. She experienced multiple chronic health conditions that were diagnosed during her medical education and she believes that her negative beliefs about her health had something to do with these conditions.

When Lissa went to the student health clinic the staff didn't seem surprised by her self-diagnoses or the other medical students coming in right before finals. The medical staff actually told her that they called this syndrome "medical student disease."

In the book, Love, Medicine & Miracles, Dr. Bernie Siegel highlights a study about patients in a control group who thought they were taking a new chemotherapy drug and warned that they could lose their hair and 30% of them lost their hair when they actually were only given saline.

An excerpt from The Scientist publication, in the article Worried Sick, published in July 2013: In New Zealand in the fall of 2007, pharmacies across the country began dispensing a new formulation of Eltroxin—the only thyroid hormone replacement drug approved and paid for by the government and used by tens of thousands of New Zealanders since 1973. Within months, reports of side effects began trickling into the government's health-care monitoring agency.

Some of the reports included known side effects of the drug, as well as symptoms not normally associated with the drug or disease. In the 18 months following the release of the new tablets, the rate of Eltroxins' adverse event reporting rose nearly 2,000.

However the active ingredient in the drug, thyroxine, was exactly the same. Laboratory testing proved that the new formulation was bioequivalent to the old one.

The only change was that the drug maker, GlaxoSmithKline, had moved its manufacturing process from Canada to Germany, and in the process altered the drug's inert qualities, such as the tablets' size, color, and markings.

So why were people getting sick? In June, it turned out, newspapers and TV stations around the country had begun to directly attribute the reported adverse effects to the changes in the drug. Following widespread coverage of the issue, more and more patients reported adverse events to the government. And the areas of the country with the most intense media coverage had the highest rates of reported ill effects, suggesting that perhaps a little social persuasion was at play.

In Napoleon Hill's book, Think and Grow Rich, he explains the power of autosuggestion which applies to all suggestions whether self-administered or continuously heard or thought about and taken in through the five senses.

When thoughts are continuously held in the conscious mind whether negative or positive they eventually seep down into the subconscious mind, (which is our operating system) and influence the subconscious mind with these positive or negative thoughts.

Once this occurs the subconscious mind goes to work and makes these thoughts your reality. So if you have a diagnosis and you research all the symptoms that could possibly happen and start looking for these symptoms you just might experience them.

When I was diagnosed with the aneurysm, I never researched anything about this condition or what could happen. I did not ask my Doctor what could happen or if anything negative could happen with the new procedure I chose instead of surgery.

I kept my mind in a blank state about the illness and actually set about believing that the aneurysm did not exist. I ran mental movies of being healthy walking on the beach and spent time looking at pictures of myself that showed me being healthy and active.

From Maxwell Maltz, Psycho-cybernetics in 1964, "If the imagination is vivid enough and detailed enough, your imagination practice is equivalent to an actual experience, insofar as your nervous system is concerned. Your nervous system cannot tell the difference between an imagined experience and a "real" experience. In either case, it reacts automatically to information which you give it from your forebrain…your nervous system reacts appropriately to what you think or imagine to be true."

Bruce H. Lipton PHD, in the book The Biology of Belief states, "thoughts, the mind's energy, directly influence how the physical brain controls the body's physiology. Harnessing the power of your mind can be more effective than the drugs you have been programmed to believe you need."

Dr. Eric Robbins, a Urologist in California, states in a video that he got tired of using medication to treat the symptoms of illness, which didn't really address the underlying problem. He also states that it's possible to clear emotional problems at a deep enough level with alternative energy healing techniques so that physical healing results.

Dr. Robbins has been using mind, body, healing techniques in his practice for over 20 years.

Helping Others Create Miraculous Healings

After the joyful experience of healing myself, I desire to help people know they have the power to improve areas in their life as well, through harnessing the power of their thoughts, impressing wellbeing upon the subconscious mind, receiving energy healing processes, and through connection to all that is, God or Higher Power.

I have created a partnership with my clients to assist them in releasing symptoms of illness, fears, worries, depression, emotional trauma, and past negative events. We work together to release core beliefs or thoughts that contribute to lack in any area of the person's life. Using these tools helps lift the energy vibration of the body, which helps the person feel calm and peaceful and begin the healing process.

Reconnective Healing, an energy healthcare process, is a return to an optimal state of balance, wholeness and vitality. It is a bridge between the perceived limitations we have come to accept in our lives and how life can be when we tap into our actual potential.

It's tangible, measurable... You can actually feel it! Reconnective Healing gives you access to an inner awareness with a vibrational resonance that promotes strength, brainpower, wisdom, emotional stability and physical vitality. When you access this spectrum of Energy, Light & Information®, it creates a chain of events that can greatly enhance and improve all aspects of your life — health, career, relationships, abundance... Seemingly unreachable potential becomes reality.

Recognized and supported by science, including researchers affiliated with institutions such as Harvard, Yale and Stanford. Reconnective Healing offers the opportunity to attain lifelong optimal health and balance.

"The cutting-edge of information medicine."

– Stanford Professor Emeritus
Dr. William Tiller

Reconnective Healing has been scientifically shown* to:

- Restructure damaged DNA
- Be more than twice as effective as physical therapy in restoring range of motion

• Support athletic peak performance

*Scientific studies are available at TheReconnection.com

The Power of Loving Support Helps Induce Healing

Kristy gave me the gift of love, friendship, and support on my journey to heal myself. She witnessed and was a part of all the laughter, joy and connection with God energy that allowed me to once again be the healthy person I had always been.

In 2013, Kristy experienced her own health challenge and she asked me to help her overcome this challenge. Kristy lived in Kentucky and I live in Florida so we conducted some sessions over the phone and we also had one session in-person when she came to Florida to visit. I used energy healing processes with Kristy to release negative feelings, emotions and images she

had stored in her mind and body regarding her health challenge.

During one of the sessions we
tapped into the subconscious mind
and were able to find the core incident
or root cause of the illness and release
the negative thoughts and feelings that
formed into the illness.

In another session, we went back
to a childhood event where we released
buried emotions that played a part in
manifesting relationships that did not
serve her.

We knew she had released the
negative feelings regarding the core
incident and childhood event when
she could talk about these events and
remember them but she no longer had
any negative emotions or negative feelings about the incidents.

We did a session to change the
way she saw herself when she looked in

the mirror because she had experienced some changes in her appearance due to the symptoms of illness. We tapped in the vision of looking in the mirror and seeing herself the way she had always been before the diagnosis.

We also recalibrated her thyroid from working at 18% effectiveness to working at 86% of effectiveness. We continued to do sessions to calibrate and maintain a high effectiveness of her thyroid while she began to feel better and lower her medication.

Kristy did energy healing process-es in-between sessions, used the ideas of the law of attraction to see herself healthy and impressed wellbeing on her subconscious mind. She knew that she had created the illness unconsciously by the events she had experienced and the negative emotions tied to these events. She began to release the symptoms of the illness and feel better. She had a blood test to check and see if the thy-roid markers matched how she was feeling. The test results showed normal ranges for her thyroid and she is now free of the symptoms of the illness. Kristy's message about healing from Graves Disease with my guidance:

I went to Sherry to get help with a chronic health issue, Graves Disease, an autoimmune thyroid disorder, that I had been diagnosed with two years earlier. I had been told by several doctors that Graves Disease is incurable and that I would need to either have surgery to remove my thyroid or have radioactive iodine treatment to destroy my thyroid, neither of which I wanted to do.

I finally found an endocrinologist who agreed to try medication to manage the disease and symptoms. My symptoms were under control when I met with Sherry, but I wanted to heal myself completely so I could stop taking the medication.

I had already changed my lifestyle and was focusing on eating a healthy diet, staying active, managing stress, and getting adequate sleep. However, it was the energy healing sessions with Sherry that allowed me to heal and wean off the medication.

As Sherry conducted the energy healing sessions, I realized, for the first time I had connected the disease with the toxic relationship I had been in at the time of diagnosis. The energy healing sessions helped me to release the negative emotions and guilt that I was holding on to. With Sherry's guidance, I was able to forgive myself and replace those negative feelings with feelings of love and understanding. I could feel that by healing myself of the emotional trauma, my body would also be healed from the disease. And all of this happened in three sessions!

I have been off of all medication for over a year now and I am perfectly healthy. I still see my endocrinologist regularly and all my thyroid markers are within normal ranges.

Sherry has a remarkable ability to connect with people and make them feel comfortable. I was completely at ease during the sessions and was amazed at her intuition to guide me so that I saw clearly things I had not thought of before. I believe that Sherry has a true gift for healing. I recommend scheduling a session with her for any disorder or problem that you want help with.

Note: Every person is a unique individual and healing may take more sessions or multiple therapies to change ingrained beliefs or to find the core incident and release it.

As always, Reconnective Healing or energy healing processes are complimentary to medical care and not a replacement for medical care.

Chapter Eight -
THE POWER OF LOVE

"Love yourself first and everything else falls into line."

-Lucille Ball

"Love is the essential reality and our purpose on earth. To be consciously aware of it, to experience love in ourselves and others, is the meaning of life. Meaning does not lie in things. Meaning lies in us."

-Marianne Williamson

You have probably heard that you can't love someone else until you love yourself first. If you think about the law of attraction which is defined as like attracts like, if you don't love yourself then you will attract someone who doesn't love their self either.

So both parties are looking for love from outside and not able to give love to their partner because you can't give what you don't have. The relationship you have with yourself effects every other relationship you have. If you love yourself others will love you.

A foundation of love was instrumental in my healing from the aneurysm. When the diagnosis came in, I went into appreciation and gratitude for everything in my life, including appreciating myself, and my connection with God.

I made time to be in laughter each day. I spent time in nature as much as I could and used self-hypnosis to let go of any stress. I asked my Doctor if I could continue my planned trip to Florida because I knew it would be beneficial for my health and well-being. I had the opportunity to explore many areas in Florida and did something fun every day. I was in a high state of joy each day.

From the book, Health Revelations from Heaven and Earth, by loving yourself, you are honoring God's gift of life. Self-Love activates the Divine Spark within you. You will become love, and you will find your life filled with miracles and possibilities. So love yourself first – without ego – and you will be complete within.

The physical body is made up of energy that operates within a vibration or frequency. The vibration of love and joy is free from ego or negative thoughts.

Steps you can take to raise your love or joy vibration:

Make a list of all the things that you appreciate about yourself and say them out loud in an enthusiastic voice, such as:

- I appreciate how kind I am to others
- I appreciate how friendly I am
- I appreciate how well I communicate
- I appreciate my commitment to exercise
- I appreciate my ability to be flexible
- I appreciate how smart I am
- I appreciate how well I parent my children
- I appreciate my ability to get things done
- I appreciate how things are always working out for me

- I appreciate my family and friends
- I love and appreciate myself

You may not believe what you are saying initially, but over time you will begin to accept these messages that are sinking down into your subconscious mind.

Other strategies to raise your vibration:

- Spend time in nature
- Meditate
- Listen to upbeat music
- Watch a funny show, something that will really give you a belly laugh
- Hold a puppy or kitten
- Observe young children playing and laughing
- Fly a kite or let a balloon go

According to Lissa Renna, MD, happy people live 7 to 10 years longer than pessimistic people and optimistic people are 77% less likely to get heart disease.

Lissa shares, if you have a negative thought, belief or feeling in the brain, the brain perceives this as a threat. If you feel lonely, have a pessimistic thought, don't like your job, have a negative thought about yourself or are in a toxic relationship, the mind perceives this as a threat and turns on the amygdala which says threat. This begins to produce chemicals and stress hormones like cortisol, noraphrine, and epinephrine.

The stress response turns on and triggers the sympathetic nervous system and puts you into the fight or flight mode, which is protective and adaptive if you are running away from a bear but is meant to be a quick stress response to solve the threat and then switch off and come back to a normal state. In modern day life we experience as many as 50 stress responses a day in traffic, at our jobs, or in our relationships.

The good news is that there is a relaxation response we can tap into, and when the relaxation response kicks in, the stress response switches off and the parasympathetic nervous system switches on and our own healing hormones are produced such as oxytocin, dopamine, nitric oxide, and endorphins, which are released in the body and bathe all the cells.

The relaxation response and healing hormones cannot be released when the body is in flight or fight mode. These natural healing processes are only available when you are in a relaxed state. So you are not receiving the healing hormones while experiencing a negative emotion or feeling stress or anxiety.

So the good thing is that you can get into the relaxation response by doing meditation or yoga; receiving a Reconnective Healing session, hypnosis session, or a massage; being in nature, doing work you love, experiencing laughter, supportive relationships, or sex.   Likewise Marilyn Mandala Schlitz, PHD, stated when you go from frustration to joy 1400 chemical changes happen in the body.

Your words are powerful and creative for yourself and those around you. Dr. Emoto wanted to show that water has emotional memory, so he did an experiment where he put distilled water in several jars and put the words thank you on one jar, hate on another jar and nothing on the third jar.

When the words "thank you" were taped to a bottle of distilled water, the frozen crystals had a similar shape to the crystals formed by water that had been exposed to Bach's "Goldberg Variations"- music composed out of gratitude to the man it was named for.

When water samples were bombarded with heavy metal music or labeled with negative words, or when negative thoughts and emotions were focused intentionally upon these samples, such as "Adolf Hitler", the water did not form crystals at all and displayed chaotic, fragmented structures.

The average adult human body is 50-65% water, averaging around 57-60%. The percentage of water in infants is much higher, typically around 75-78% water, then dropping to 65% by one year of age.

When we change our words, thoughts, and environment from negative to positive, it affects our life and everyone and everything around us.

The result was that beautiful crystals formed after giving the water good words, playing good music, and offering pure prayer to water. Disfigured crystals occurred when negative words or loud disruptive music was played.

In the book, The Power of the Subconscious Mind, by Joseph Murphy, he states, "Love is the fulfilling of the law of health, happiness, and peace of mind."

Living life from a state of love for yourself and love for the life you are creating is a powerful way to live. I believe that being in a state of joy, love, and appreciation, surrounded by people that loved me and connected with God energy, healed me.

About the Author -

Sherry is a Wellness Coach in the energy psychology field. She is a Reconnective Healing Foundational Practitioner, Certified Hypnotherapist, Heart to Heart Tapping Meditation Practitioner, and holds a certificate in Care Ministry. Sherry is also certified as a Global Career Development Facilitator, Professional in Human Resources and has a Bachelor's Degree in Psychology. Sherry has 22 years of experience in the Human Resource Management field.

Sherry's passion is to help her clients live their best life and return to an optimal state of balance, and therefore an optimal state of health and evolution.

The effects of a healing session may be felt on the physical, mental, emotional, and spiritual levels.

Sherry lives in Palm Beach Gardens, Florida.

Sherry's website:
www.efthealingfl.com
Email: emotional-freedom@live.com

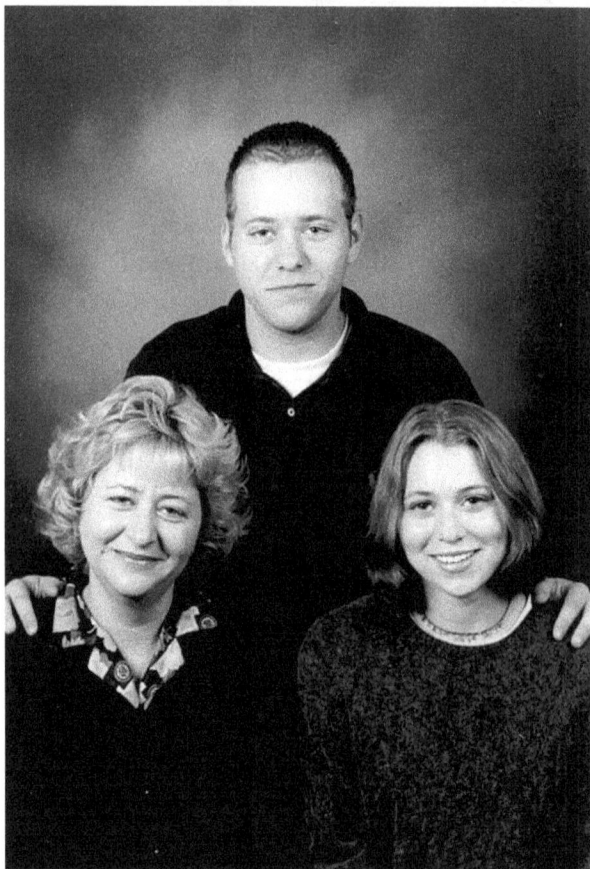